Paleo Italian Cookbook

Healthy, Delicious, Low Carb and Gluten Free Recipes

Table of Contents

About the Book

This book is full of delicious and healthy Italian recipes for followers of the Paleo diet. Learn more about the Paleo diet in the introduction. Then explore the flavors and combinations of Italian style cooking that are made to be delicious appetizers, breakfast recipes, lunch recipes, dinner recipes and last but certainly not least, desserts! Enjoy the collection of delicious & nutritious meals, desserts & snacks while getting into your Paleo habits.

About the Book

Introduction

The Paleolithic diet is a way of eating from 10,000 years ago in the Paleolithic era, also known as the caveman diet, Stone Age diet & hunter gatherer diet. It consists of foods that were eaten before the agricultural revolution and wheat-based diet developed. These diets consist of meat, seafood, fruits, vegetables and nuts. All foods that are in their natural form, not processed and wheat-free are included. Studies are showing that human bodies are better adapted to this way of eating.

Foods in their natural form contain a great deal of vitamins and minerals. By including these in daily eating, many health benefits may be achieved. Many of the traditional recipes that people love, have a Paleo version that are just as delicious, if not more so. An added bonus is you are giving your body the nutrients it needs, so there is no guilt. Best of luck on your journey eating clean with Paleo! These recipes can be a starting point to help you create new favorite meals. Following the Paleo diet, people have found the following health benefits:-

- A healthy body weight
- Lowered cholesterol
- Decreased high blood pressure
- Decreased cardiac problems
- Experienced increased energy
- Lower cancer risks
- Reduce allergies
- Improves respiratory problems such as asthma
- Stabilized blood sugar levels

Now, let's have a little chat about the Italian cuisine. Italian cuisine is famous around the world for its richness & diversity. Typically prepared with fresh ingredients from recipes spanning generations; Italian food is a basic element of Italian heritage & one of the country's core cultural exports. Restaurants serve Italian food in just about every international city. Italian cookbooks can be found in almost any bookstore. While many people associate Italian food with a few standard dishes like pizza, spaghetti and lasagna, there is actually terrific diversity among the various regional cuisines of Italy. The history of Italian cuisine could be an entire book by itself, but this book is your starting point to Paleo Italian foods. Many think Italian dishes are out of the picture when they start the Paleo diet, but it does not have to be the case! Find out more as you taste your way through this book.

Appetizer

Paleo Italian Meatballs

22 Servings

Cook time: 20 minutes

1 lb. ground beef

3 links fresh Paleo Italian Sausage (mild or hot)

1 small onion (finely diced)

2 garlic cloves (minced)

3 tbsp. almond meal

2 tbsp. flax seed meal

1 tbsp. chopped herbs, to taste (thyme parsley, oregano)

3 eggs

1 tsp. sea salt

1 tsp. black pepper

Take a large bowl; add & combine all the ingredients until well mixed. Scoop & roll the meatballs and then, pan fry or bake at 350 degrees for about 16 to 20 minutes, or until cooked through. Finally, serve them with your favorite sauce & spaghetti squash.

Salmon Carpaccio

4 Servings

Cook time: 2 minutes

4 oz. smoked salmon

1/4 c. extra-virgin olive oil

1 tbsp. red onion (minced)

2 tbsp. lemon juice

1 tbsp. Italian parsley (minced)

2 tbsp. capers

Sea salt & black pepper (to taste)

First; thinly slice the smoked salmon into strips. Then, place them in a small mixing bowl. Next, add in the remaining ingredients; gently toss together & serve with your favorite sauce.

Italian Stuffed Eggs

4-8 Servings

Cook time: 0 minutes

4 large hard-boiled eggs (peeled & sliced in half laterally)

3 tbsp. olive oil

1 ½ tsp. onions (finely minced)

1 tsp. garlic (finely minced)

1/8 tsp. ground black pepper

1 tbsp. fresh basil leaves (finely chopped)

1 tbsp. fresh Italian parsley, flat leaf (finely chopped)

Paprika

First; remove the egg yolks from the whites. Then, place the egg whites cut side up onto a plate. Next, in a small bowl; add & mash the egg yolks with a fork. Stir in 1 tablespoon of olive oil, onion, garlic & black pepper. Then, stir in the basil & parsley. Now, gradually add in the remaining olive oil; stir until smooth. Adjust the seasoning & add in additional black pepper (if desired). Finally, spoon the egg yolks mixture into the egg white halves and sprinkle with the paprika.

Marinated Italian Mushrooms

8 Servings

Cook time: 0 minutes

8 oz. mushrooms (cleaned & quartered)

4 tbsp. fresh lemon juice

1/4 c. olive oil

2 tbsp. fresh parsley (finely chopped)

1/4 tsp. tarragon

Sea salt & pepper (to taste)

Take a mixing bowl; add & combine all the ingredients. Mix them well. Then add in the mushrooms; mix well again. Next, cover & refrigerate for about 24 hours. Serve and enjoy!

Paleo Italian, Almond Cookies (Chocolate Dipped)

14 Servings

Cook time: 20 minutes

2 c. slivered almonds or whole (if skinless)

1 c. organic coconut sugar

2 egg (just the whites)

1 tsp. raw almond extract

1/2 tsp. vanilla extract

1/8 tsp. sea salt (optional)

1 tbsp. sliced almond (optional)

2 tbsp. dark chocolate chips (optional)

Pre-heat the oven to 300 degrees & line a baking sheet with parchment paper. Take a food processor; add & grind the almond slivers into a fine meal. Next, add in the coconut sugar & process for about 15 seconds more. Add in the whites of 2 eggs, extract of almonds and vanilla & sea salt; make it into a paste. Now, place the processor bowl into a freezer for about 7 minutes. After freezing, spoon it onto parchment paper and garnish with the almond slices (optional). Place into the oven & bake for about 20 to 30 minutes, or until golden. Remove & let them cool completely before removing from the baking sheet. Melt the chocolate & drizzle on ¼ portion of each cookie (optional). Place the cookies into the freezer for a few minute to help the chocolate dry faster.

Breakfast

Egg Breakfast Chili

5 Servings

Cook time: 30 minutes

1 lb. ground beef

1/2 onion (finely diced)

8 oz. tomatoes (crushed)

3 c. beef stock

1 small sweet potato (peeled & diced)

1 tbsp. paprika

1 tbsp. granulated garlic

2 tsp. chili powder

1 tsp. onion powder

2 tbsp. lime juice

2 tbsp. hot sauce

2 tsp. smoked paprika

Sea salt (to taste)

4 eggs

1/4 avocado

First, sauté the meat in a soup pot and then, fry the onions until cooked well. Add in the potatoes, tomatoes & spices; let it simmer for about 20 minutes or until the potatoes cooked through. Next, scramble an egg for every person; serve in a bowl with chili. Top with scrambled egg, a few bacon & avocado slices.

Paleo Breakfast Casserole

8 Servings

Cook time: 45 minutes

18 eggs

1 c. red onion (chopped)

2 c. fresh mushrooms, sliced

1 1/2 c. yellow squash (chopped)

2 c. butternut squash or zucchini (chopped)

3 c. fresh baby spinach

10 strips bacon, cooked

Sea salt, pepper & garlic powder (to taste)

Pre-heat the oven to 350 degrees. Take a large bowl; add & combine all the ingredients; stir well to combine. Add in the garlic powder, salt & pepper (to taste). Then, grease bottom & sides of a 9x13 inches baking dish with a little coconut oil. Next, pour all ingredients from bowl into the baking dish. Place in oven & bake for about 45 minutes.

Paleo Delicious Hash Browns

2 Servings

Cook time: 30 minutes

1 spaghetti squash

1 onion (finely diced)

2 tsp. chopped rosemary

2 tbsp. olive oil

Pre-heat the oven to 450 degrees. Divide the spaghetti squash into half & remove the seeds. Lightly spread some olive oil into the hollow space of the squash & lay it downward onto the baking sheet. Bake for about 20 minutes; turn the side over & roast for another 20 minutes. Then, take out from oven & let it cool for some time. While the squash is baking; heat up some olive oil on medium high heat in a saucepan, add in the sliced onion & rosemary. Next, place the squash in a bowl; add in the onions & mix roughly to combine. Turn the flame to high heat; add oil to frying pan (if needed). Take a ladle, spoon up some squash mix; fry it till caramelized & golden brown for about 10 minutes on each side. Repeat the same until all done.

Paleo Crispy Coconut Macaroons

3 Servings

Cook time: 45 minutes

1/2 c. egg whites

1/4 c. honey

1/4 tsp. sea salt

1 c. unsweetened coconut (finely shredded)

Pre-heat the oven to 200 degrees and line a baking sheet with parchment paper. Take a blender, or food processor; add & blend egg whites, salt, and honey on high speed for about 5 minutes, or until stiff crests have formed. Next, add in the coconut & whip to combine. Place the macaroon into a zip top plastic bag & zip tightly. Now, cut off one tip of the bag and squeeze the bag to form circle shapes onto the baking sheet. Bake in the oven till crisp & browned. Enjoy!

Paleo Breakfast Skillet

5 Servings

Cook time: 45 minutes

1 lb. Paleo breakfast sausage

1 large sweet potato (diced)

5 eggs

1 avocado (diced)

Handful of cilantro

Hot sauce (to taste)

Raw cheese (optional)

Pre-heat the oven to 400 degrees. Take an oven safe pan, break & brown the sausage on medium high heat. Once browned, remove the sausage & allow it cool for some time. Then, transfer the potatoes into the sausage oil & allow them get brittle & cooked. Add the sausage to the pan; make wells in the pan, one for each egg. Crack the eggs into the wells; place the skillet into the oven & bake for about 5 minutes, or until the yolks are cooked through. Remove from the oven; cover the top with avocado, cilantro & hot sauce. Serve one egg per person, along with its adjacent goodies.

Pizza Stuffed Sweet Potatoes

5 Servings

Cook time: 50 minutes

4 sweet potatoes

8 oz. mushrooms (sliced)

2 black olives (sliced)

1 lb. freshly ground beef

1 onion (thinly sliced0

Pizza toppings

For the Sauce

2 c. tomato sauce

2 tsp. olive oil

1 tbsp. onion powder

1 tbsp. dried oregano

2 tsp. garlic powder

Pre-heat the oven to 400 degrees. Pierce & then place the sweet potatoes on a baking sheet; let them sauté for about 40 minutes or until soft & soggy. In the meantime, stir together the sauce items, taste & adjust the seasoning, then set it aside. Then, in a large frying pan, crush & brown the beef. Remove the meat from the pan, toss in mushrooms, & onions; let them cook until the mushrooms are browned & the onions are spongy. Once the potatoes are done, slice them & place the pieces onto the baking sheet. Smash the sweet potatoes insides with a splitter, then, scoop a few dollops of sauce onto the potatoes, followed by the onion, mushrooms, olives & sausage. Bake for about 2 to 3 minutes to warm-up & serve.

Lunch

Paleo Italian Seafood Stew

6 Servings

Cook time: 30 minutes

1 lb firm white fish (Cod, Haddock or Mahi Mahi)

1 dozen medium or large shrimp (shelled)

1/2 lb. squid rings (& tentacles if desired)

1 dozen fresh mussels or clams (cleaned)

3 tbsp. olive oil

1 medium red onion (diced)

1 red or green bell pepper (diced)

4 garlic cloves (diced)

2 tbsp. fresh parsley (diced)

2 c. fresh chopped tomatoes or 14 oz diced tomatoes with juices

2 tsp. smoked paprika

1 tsp. crushed red pepper (to taste)

1 tsp. sea salt (to taste)

Freshly ground black pepper (to taste)

4 c. chicken stock

Take a saucepan; add olive oil & heat on medium-high heat. Add in the onion, bell pepper, garlic & parsley; sauté until the onion becomes translucent; stir occasionally. Then, add in the chopped tomatoes, smoked paprika, red pepper flakes, salt & pepper; sauté for 5 additional minutes. Next, add in the squid (optional) & let it simmer for about 5 minutes. Now, add in all the remaining seafood & the stock; gently stir to combine. Bring the pan up to a strong simmer & cover it for about 15 minutes. Once, the mussels and/or clams have opened; remove the pan from the heat & gently ladle the stew into serving bowls.

Cabbage Salad

6 Servings

Cook time: 5 minutes

4 c. green cabbage (finely shredded)

1 medium apple (diced)

1 c. pomegranate seeds

1 c. golden raisins

1/4 c. extra-virgin olive oil

2 tbsp. lemon juice

Sea salt & pepper (to taste)

Take a large mixing bowl; add & combine the green cabbage, apple, pomegranate seeds & golden raisins; mix them well. Then, in another small mixing bowl; whisk together the extra-virgin olive oil & lemon juice. Next, drizzle the dressing over the salad & toss together. Finally, season with salt & pepper (to taste); enjoy!

Italian Meatloaf

3-4 Servings

Cook time: 40 minutes

For the meatloaf

1 lb. grass-fed ground beef

1 yellow onion (diced)

1 roasted red pepper (diced)

1/4 c. tomato sauce

1 egg (whisked)

3/4 c. almond flour

1 tsp. dried basil

1 tsp. dried thyme

1 tsp. dried parsley

Sea salt & pepper (to taste)

Olive oil (for frying)

For the sauce

3/4 c. tomato sauce

1 tsp. dried basil

1 tsp. dried thyme

1 tsp. dried parsley

Sea salt & pepper (to taste)

Fresh basil, chopped (optional)

Pre-heat the oven to 400 degrees. Place a skillet onto medium-high heat, add in 1 to 2 tablespoon of oil, onions & roasted red pepper to the pot. Sauté until onions turn soft & translucent. Once ready, add them into a large bowl, along with the remaining ingredients; mix well with your hands. Next, place the dough into a bread pan & bake for about 40 minutes. Once, meatloaf is ready, add sausage ingredients to a pan to heat up slightly, until bubbly. Let the meatloaf cool slightly & top with sauce. Finally, top with fresh basil & eat it up!

Italian Crock Pot Chili

6-8 Servings

Cook time: 6 hours

3-4 lb. freshly ground beef

1 onion (chopped)

10 oz. mushrooms (diced)

28 oz. tomatoes (fire-roasted)

1 tbsp. garlic (minced)

3-4 tbsp. capers

1/4 small can of tomato paste

1-2 c. stock or broth

3 bay leaves

2 tbsp. dried thyme

2 tbsp. dried basil

2 tbsp. chili powder

1 tbsp. cayenne (optional)

Sea salt & pepper (to taste)

2-3 tbsp. balsamic vinegar

Olive oil (for spray)

First; put the ground beef in the crock pot, along with salt, pepper & diced onion; trim the flame & sauté for about 3 hours, stirring occasionally. Then, drain and toss the meat back; add in the tomato paste, mushrooms, garlic, capers, and tomatoes; stir to combine well. Next, add in the rest of the ingredients to make chili & mix well. Cook it on low heat for about 3 hours or until the veggies are ready.

Balsamic 'Brown Sugar' Chicken

3-4 Servings

Cook time: 40 minutes

4 chicken breasts (boneless)

2 tbsp. ghee

2 garlic cloves (minced)

1/4 c. brown sugar or coconut sugar

2 tbsp. balsamic vinegar

Sea salt & black pepper (to taste)

Pre-heat the oven to 400 degrees. Place a small pan on medium-low heat; melt the ghee, brown sugar or coconut sugar & balsamic vinegar. Then, add in the garlic & stir to combine well. Now, place the chicken breasts into a baking dish and cover with the prepared mixture. Finally, season it with salt & black pepper (to taste). Place in the oven & bake, un-covered, for about 30 minutes, or until the chicken is cooked well.

Dinner

Meatballs with Spinach

6 Servings

Cook time: 15 minutes

2 lb. fresh ground beef

2 egg yolks

2 c. spinach (finely chopped)

4 garlic cloves (minced)

2 tbsp. fresh sage (minced)

2 tsp. sea salt

1 tsp. black pepper

4-6 tbsp. olive oil or ghee (for frying)

Take a large bowl; add & combine the beef, egg yolks, spinach, garlic, sage, salt & pepper; mix them well. Then, shape the meat mixture into meatballs slightly larger than a golf ball. Next, in a large skillet; heat the olive oil or ghee on medium heat. Place the meatballs into the skillet & sauté until evenly browned on all sides. Now, cover the meatballs; lower the heat and let it cook covered for about 7-10 minutes more, or until they are done all the way through. Serve with your favorite paleo sauce.

Italian Herb Roast Chicken

4-5 Servings

Cook time: 70 minutes

4-5 lb whole chicken

Sea salt (to taste)

Freshly ground black pepper (to taste)

2 tbsp. fresh basil

2 tbsp. fresh parsley

2 tbsp. fresh thyme

2 tbsp. fresh oregano

2 springs rosemary (chopped)

1/4 c. olive oil

1 lemon (halved)

2 bay leaves

3 sprigs of fresh rosemary

Pre-heat the oven to 400 degrees. Rinse the chicken with water & pat dry with paper towels. Take a small bowl; add & combine basil, parsley, thyme, oregano and rosemary together. Sprinkle inside of chicken cavity with sea salt. Then, grasp the skin at the tip of the chicken breast & gently pull up. Carefully, with the fingers gently separate the skin from the breast meat; try not to tear the skin. Next, sprinkle a little salt into the gaps & spread chopped herb mixture; drizzle with a little olive oil. Now, stuff the cavity with the lemon, bay leaves, rosemary springs & any residual herbs. Pull the skin of chicken breast over the breast so that none of the meat is exposed. Tuck in the wings & truss with kitchen string. Rub some olive oil onto the chicken & sprinkle with salt and pepper. Spray some oil into the roasting pan & place the chicken on one side, breast side down, and put it back in the oven. Bake for about 5 minutes, then turn the chicken and cook for another 5 minutes. Then turn the chicken over so that it is back-side down. Cook for about 1 hour, or until the juices run clear (not pink) when a knife tip is inserted into both the chicken breast and thigh.

Paleo Italian Pasta Sauce

10 Servings

Cook time: 6 hours

1 lb. pork neck bones

3 lb. paleo sausage (Italian)

3 lb. paleo meatballs (cooked)

29 oz. tomato sauce

15 oz. tomato paste

8 oz. dry red wine

4 garlic cloves (minced)

4 tbsp. oregano

4 tbsp. basil

2 tbsp. rosemary

2 tbsp. thyme

2 bay leaves

Olive oil

First, in a large saucepan; add & fry the pork-neck bones & garlic with the olive oil. Then, add in the tomato sauce, all spices, sausage (sliced into 2" parts), red wine, & tomato paste; sauté for about 6 hours on low heat, keep stirring every 30 minutes. Add in the cooked meatballs during the last 2 hours. Place the bay leaves in the sauce when served.

Salad with Italian Chicken

3-4 Servings

Cook time: 2 hrs

3-4 skinless chicken breasts (boneless)

1-2 c. Italian dressing

Salad greens (of choice)

Grated parmesan cheese (optional)

Firstly, slice the chicken breasts into strips and place them into a glass pot, cover up with Italian salad dressing and let it marinate for about 2 to 4 hours. In the meantime, prepare the salad greens. Once ready, pre-heat a steel skillet over medium-high heat and place the chicken in it; add in the salt (to taste). Next, sauté the chicken until evenly browned on all sides, keep turning occasionally. Serve instantly over greens & garnish with parmesan cheese (optional).

Crispy Italian Chicken Thighs

3-4 Servings

Cook time: 40 minutes

1 lb. chicken thighs (bone-in)

1 tbsp. garlic powder

1 tsp. red pepper flakes

1 tsp. dried oregano

1 tsp. sea salt

Pre-heat the oven to 400 degrees. Line a baking sheet with parchment paper, or foil. Take a small bowl; add & combine the garlic powder, oregano, red pepper flakes and salt. Next, place the chicken thighs onto the baking sheet, dry the skin with a paper towel & flip the thighs over so that the skin side is down. Drizzle equally with half of the seasonings on one side, turn and season the other surface. Place them in the oven and bake for about 30 minutes, or until the thighs are cooked completely.

Paleo Italian Style Chicken Rissoles

3-4 Servings

Cook time: 25 minutes

1 lb. chicken (minced)

1 brown onion (finely chopped)

1 carrot (peeled & grated)

1 tsp. oregano

1 tsp. basil

1/2 tsp. thyme

1 tbs. tomato paste

1 egg

Sea salt & pepper (to taste)

Coconut oil (to grease)

First; put all the ingredients into a bowl & mix well. Roll the minced chicken with your hands & split into 12 balls. Heat up the coconut oil in a frying pan on medium high heat. Next, place the rissoles into the pot, blend a little & cook for about 7 to 8 minutes or until golden browned. Serve with roasted vegetables & salad.

Desserts & Snacks

Paleo Coconut Mocha

5 Servings
Cook time: 30 minutes
4 c. coconut milk
1/2 c. cocoa powder
1 tsp. vanilla extract
1 tsp. coffee powder
1/4 tsp. sea salt

Firstly, put all the ingredients in a pan on the low flame. The cocoa powder won't melt till the milk has warmed up, so give it some time. Whisk it to whirl all the ingredients and serve warm, like coffee.

Paleo Cauliflower Spicy Hummus

4 Servings

Cook time: 25 minutes

4 c. steamed cauliflower

2 tbsp. tahini

5 tbsp. extra virgin olive oil

2 tbsp. Lemon juice

1 tbsp. cumin

Sea salt & pepper (to taste)

First; blend the cauliflower, tahini, lemon juice & cumin. Taste it, add some extra cumin or olive oil (if needed). You can also add some lemon juice & olive oil. Sprinkle some pepper, salt (to taste) and serve with veggies to dip.

Cumin Flavored, Baked Lotus Chips

3 Servings

Cook time: 30 minutes

1/2 lb. lotus root sliced

2 tbsp. extra virgin olive oil

1 tsp. sesame oil

2 tsp. cumin

1 tsp. curry powder

3/4 tsp. sea salt

1/2 tsp. black pepper

1/8 tsp. cinnamon

Pre-heat the oven to 350 degrees. Dip the lotus root in icy water for about 30 minutes, then drain & dry out. Then, place the wedged lotus root & oils into a mixing bowl; mix together until well mixed. Add in the left over ingredients; continue to mix together and place the chips onto a baking sheet in a layer. Bake the chips for about 20 minutes or until golden browned. Place the chips onto a wire rack to cool thoroughly & serve.

Spicy Parsnip Wedges

2 Servings

Cook time: 20 minutes

3 large parsnips sliced

1/2 tsp. sea salt

1/2 tsp. black pepper

3 tbsp. coconut oil

1/2 tsp. cumin

1 tsp. paprika

1/4 tsp. cayenne pepper

1 garlic clove (minced)

Place the parsnip slices into a bowl, mix over the coconut oil & stir until well coated. Spread the remaining ingredients & stir to combine well. Pour into a greased tray, bake at 400 degrees for about 30 minutes or until soft & golden.

Baked Yucca Fries

1 Serving

Cook time: 30 minutes

1 yucca root

1 tab. olive oil

1 tsp. sea salt

1 tsp. red pepper

1 tsp. black pepper

Pre-heat the oven to 440 degrees. Fully strip & wash the Yucca. Slice in half, further cut the stalks that are going down the groove, out of the root, then, chop up into little spears. Place the chopped Yucca onto a baking sheet. Then, sprinkle the olive oil & the left over ingredients. Place in oven & bake for about 15 minutes or until browned; serve warm.

Easy Almond Cheese

3 Servings

Cook time: 35 minutes

1 c. soaked almonds

3/4 c. water

2 tbsp. olive oil

3 tbsp. lemon juice

1 garlic clove

Pinch of Himalayan Salt

First, put all the ingredients in a food processor & process until soft. It will take some time, don't hurry. Put the nut mixture into a strainer lined with cheese cloth. Give a squeeze & put into the refrigerator for the night to set. The next morning, place it into the dehydrator for about 6 to 7 hours at 116 degrees, to form a crust.

Paleo Pizza Bites

3 Servings

Cook time: 30 minutes

5-7 oz. large pepperoni (preservative free)

2 tsp. paleo pizza sauce

2 cheese slices (optional)

2 tsp. black olives

1 tbsp. bell peppers

½ oz. mushrooms

1/2 green onions

1 tsp. deli ham

1 fresh pineapple

Pre-heat the oven to 390 degrees. Put the pepperoni on a baking sheet & place into the oven for about 9 minutes; turn them over once. In the meantime, prepare your toppings. Remove the pepperonis from the oven & place a spoon of pizza sauce on every pepperoni piece & top with ingredients. Put them again into the oven for about 10 minute or until toppings get hot & soften.

www.ingramcontent.com/pod-product-compliance
Lightning Source LLC
Chambersburg PA
CBHW080351290526
45791CB00009BA/2835